STUNNING FACTS

KU-090-189

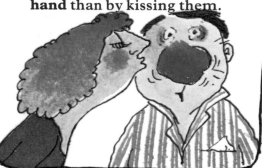

You are more likely to catch a cold by **holding** a person's **hand** than by kissing them.

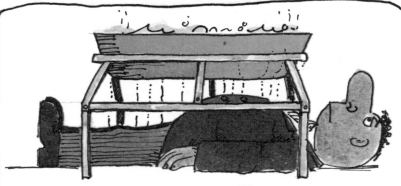

The average man produces enough heat **to boil 48 quarts** of freezing water.

Blond beards **grow faster** than dark beards.

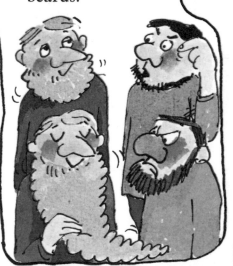

AMAZING FACTS about THE BODY

ILLUSTRATED BY BOBBIE CRAIG

Chinese and Japanese babies are born with **blue marks** on their bottoms. As they grow older the marks disappear.

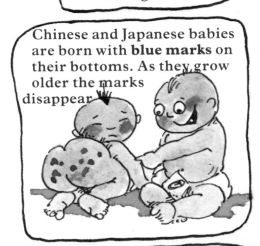

People who keep caged birds, like canaries, are **more likely** to suffer from **heart disease** than other people.

Women suffer from **chilblains more** than men.

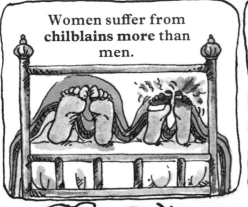

5 month old babies can tell the difference between **happy** and **angry** faces.

Hospital surveys show that new born

The chances of a mother giving birth to **quadruplets** are about 1 in 600,000

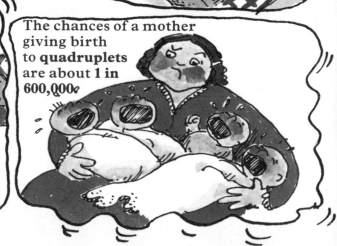

More than **15 tons** of aspirin are swallowed in America alone each year.

babies spend **133 minutes a day** crying.

THE CELL

If almost any part of a plant or animal is examined under a microscope it will be seen that it is made up of distinct units. We call these units **cells**. Since cells are too small to be seen by the human eye, they have to be magnified at least 100 times, and often more in the case of the smallest ones.

Cells come in all shapes and sizes because of the variety of jobs they have to do. Some cells are round, others look like discs and some look like rods.

Cells are grouped together to form **tissue. Tissue is gathered into groups to form organs, bones, muscles, nerves, skin, hair and every other part of the human body**.

Every second, millions of cells **die**, but through a process of existing cells **dividing**, each to make **2** new cells, millions of duplicates are **born** at the same time. Fat cells reproduce fairly slowly, but skin cells reproduce every **10** hours. The only cells in the body that are **not** replaced are brain cells, but we are born with a surplus of brain cells to make up for this continual loss.

Each cell is something like a **city** in its structure and functions. It produces the **energy** it requires in minute sausage-shaped power stations called **mitochondria**. These mitochondria burn fuel (sugar) to produce the energy the cell requires, and they leave behind water and carbon-dioxide as waste products.

The center of the cell is the **nucleus** where the cell's information is stored. Here all the instructions which the cell needs to live and work are housed.

The cell not only manufactures and stores substances, it also contains **enzymes** (chemicals) that destroy harmful particles and any old parts of the cell.

The **outer-membrane** is like a city wall, protecting the cell from harmful substances outside, it allows useful ones to enter. Waste materials made by the cell are allowed to pass out through the membrane.

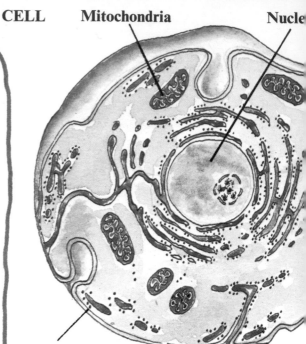

CELL   **Mitochondria**   **Nucle**

Outer Membrane

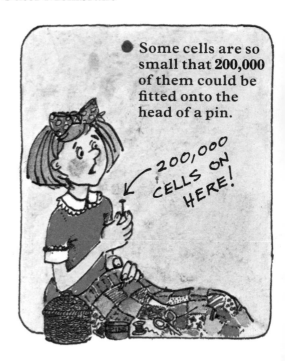

● Some cells are so small that **200,000** of them could be fitted onto the head of a pin.

200,000 CELLS ON HERE!

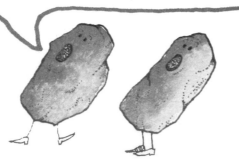

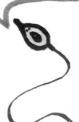

● The average size of most cells in the human body is **.0004–.0012** inches.

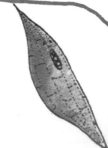

● There are about **60,000,000,000,00** cells in the human body.

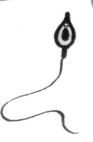

THE CELL AS A CITY

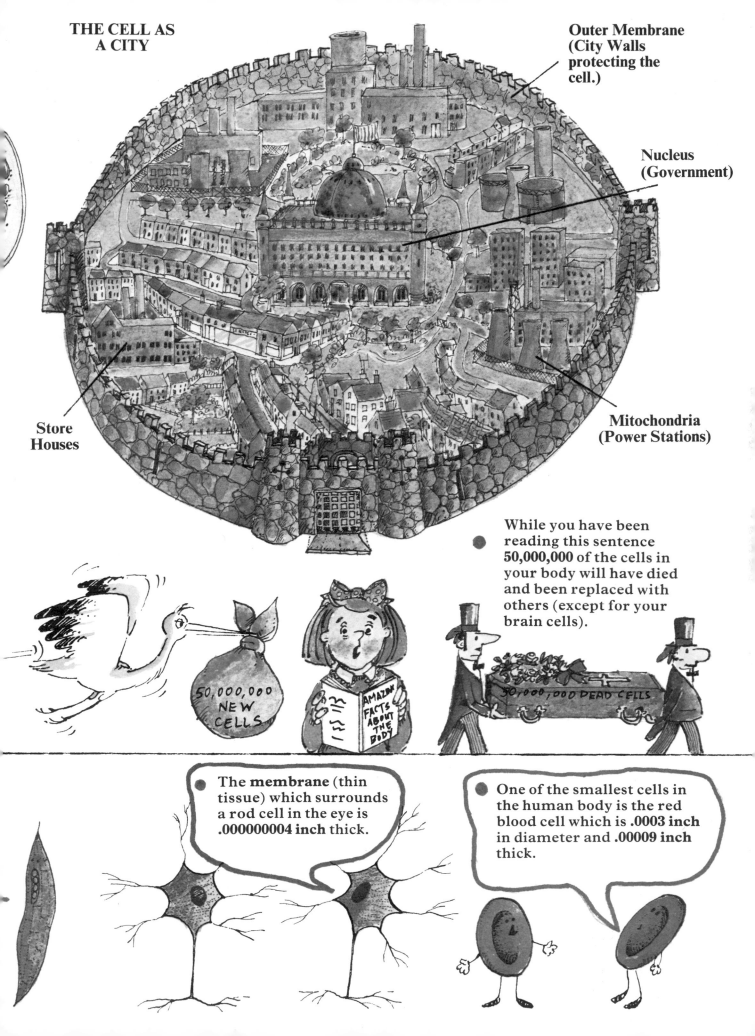

Outer Membrane (City Walls protecting the cell.)

Nucleus (Government)

Mitochondria (Power Stations)

Store Houses

While you have been reading this sentence **50,000,000** of the cells in your body will have died and been replaced with others (except for your brain cells).

50,000,000 NEW CELLS

AMAZING FACTS ABOUT THE BODY

50,000,000 DEAD CELLS

The **membrane** (thin tissue) which surrounds a rod cell in the eye is **.000000004 inch** thick.

One of the smallest cells in the human body is the red blood cell which is **.0003 inch** in diameter and **.00009 inch** thick.

THE SKELETON

The frame of bones in our bodies is called the **skeleton**.

The skeleton serves several purposes:
* *the bones give the body its general **shape**;
* *they **support** and **protect** the softer parts of the body;
* *they provide **leverage** for the fibrous tissues called
* ***muscles** that are attached to them.

Inside the hard, outer material of our bones there is a soft, yellowish substance called **marrow**. The marrow is a **supply point** for many of the important materials which we need in order to live.

Bone marrow **manufactures** some of the elements in our blood, as well as **destroying** those old elements that are no longer needed. It is a **store house** for fat, and it **stores** and **supplies** important minerals called **calcium** and **phosphorus**, which are needed to maintain a balanced, healthy body.

Bones are held together by a strong, springy tissue called **cartilage**. Cartilage also joins the bones of the **spinal column** which runs down our backs. Because cartilage is springy, it acts as a **shock absorber**. In the case of the spinal column, the cartilage **protects** the brain from being constantly jolted by the shocks which are received by the lower part of the body when we walk, run or even sit down.

The point at which bones meet is called a **joint**. There are **2** types of joint:
* *those at which the bones that meet do **not** move
* *those around which the bones **can** move freely.

The part of the skull which encloses the brain is made up of bones joined by these **immovable joints**. It is called the **cranium**. Try and work out for yourself where there are movable joints in your body. Which are the ones you move most?

At those joints where there is movement, the bones are bound together by strong fibrous tissue called **ligaments**. These tissues form thick cords attached to each bone. At least one of these cords has a small hollow that contains a fluid which **lubricates** the joint, allowing the bones to move smoothly, like parts of a machine that move smoothly because they have been lubricated by oil or grease.

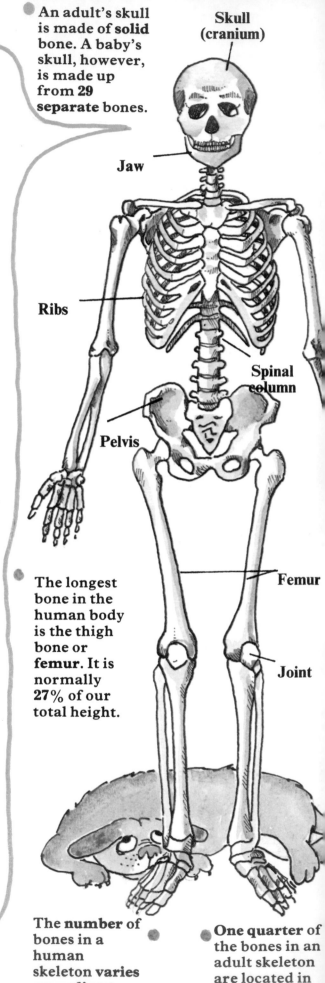

An adult's skull is made of **solid bone**. A baby's skull, however, is made up from **29 separate** bones.

Skull (cranium)

Jaw

Ribs

Spinal column

Pelvis

Femur

Joint

The longest bone in the human body is the thigh bone or **femur**. It is normally **27%** of our total height.

The **number of** bones in a human skeleton **varies according to age**.

One quarter of the bones in an adult skeleton **are located in the feet**.

BONES

The **smallest** bone is the **stirrup** bone in the middle ear. It is between **.1** and **.14 inch** long.

There is only **one** bone in our body that does not meet up with any other. It is called the **hyoid** and is in the throat.

Bones are **made** in different ways according to their **size** and **shape**.

LONG BONES

Long bones are usually made of a long cylindrical shaft with larger, thicker ends which are shaped to fit the bones to which they are connected.

SHORT BONES

Short bones, like the ones found in our wrists and ankles, are made of soft material covered with a thin layer of harder bone.

FLAT BONES

Flat bones, like the ribs consist of **2 plates** of **1in** hard bone with a softer material set between them.

Babies are usually born with about **350** separate bones.

As babies grow many bones **join** together to form larger, single bones.

A fully grown adult usually has **206** bones.

Some people have a couple of **extra** bones, as some of their bones did not grow properly together. Others have a couple **less** as more bones grow together.

The **thigh** bone is the **strongest** bone in the human body. Measured ounce for ounce it can withstand greater pressure and support a greater weight than a rod of the same size made of **solid steel**.

The **tallest** recorded height of a man was **8ft 11 inch**. His thigh bone was **2.5 feet** long.

$2\frac{1}{2}$ ft.

The horse has only **one** less bone on average than man, although it can carry a **man** on its back with no difficulty.

The cartilage in the spinal column gets squashed when we are upright, and expands when we lie down, so in the morning you are about a **quarter of an inch** taller than the night before.

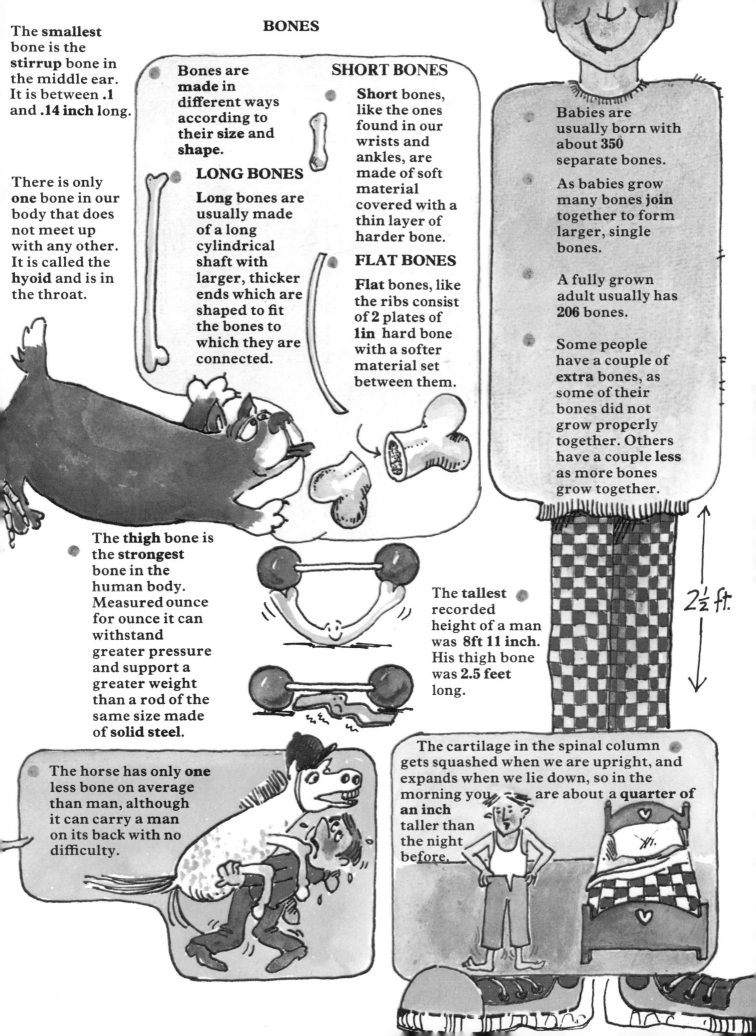

MUSCLES

The bones in our bodies have no way of moving on their own. All our movement is the work of **muscles**.

Muscles are made of fibrous tissues bound together, and they act like bunches of rubber bands.

The ends of muscles are **attached to** bones. One end is attached to a bone that the muscle is intended to **move**. The other end is anchored to a bone that the muscles will **not** move. the muscle is usually attached to the bone by a short, tough cord called a **tendon**. Tendons are made from the same kind of tissue from which ligaments are made.

There are **2** kinds of muscles in the body. The ones that we can move at will are called **voluntary** muscles. Those that we cannot move as we wish are called **involuntary** muscles. Some examples of involuntary muscles are: those that allow us to move our eyes; the ones that control our tongue and soft palate. Involuntary muscles are also found in the walls of our intestines, stomach, veins and arteries.

There are over **3** times as many muscles in the adult body as there are bones; around **656** altogether.

Muscles are heavy. They make up about **42%** of a man's body weight and about **36%** of a woman's weight.

Muscles can only work in **one** way, by **pulling**. They never work by pushing. The muscle system in your body is arranged so that even if you are pushing against something with all your strength, your muscles are all really **pulling**.

17 SMILING MUSCLES

You use **17** muscles to smile and **43** to frown.

The largest muscle in your body is the one in your **buttock** which extends your thigh bone

One of the muscles in the region of your nose and upper lip has the name 'lefator labii superioris aloequae nasi'.

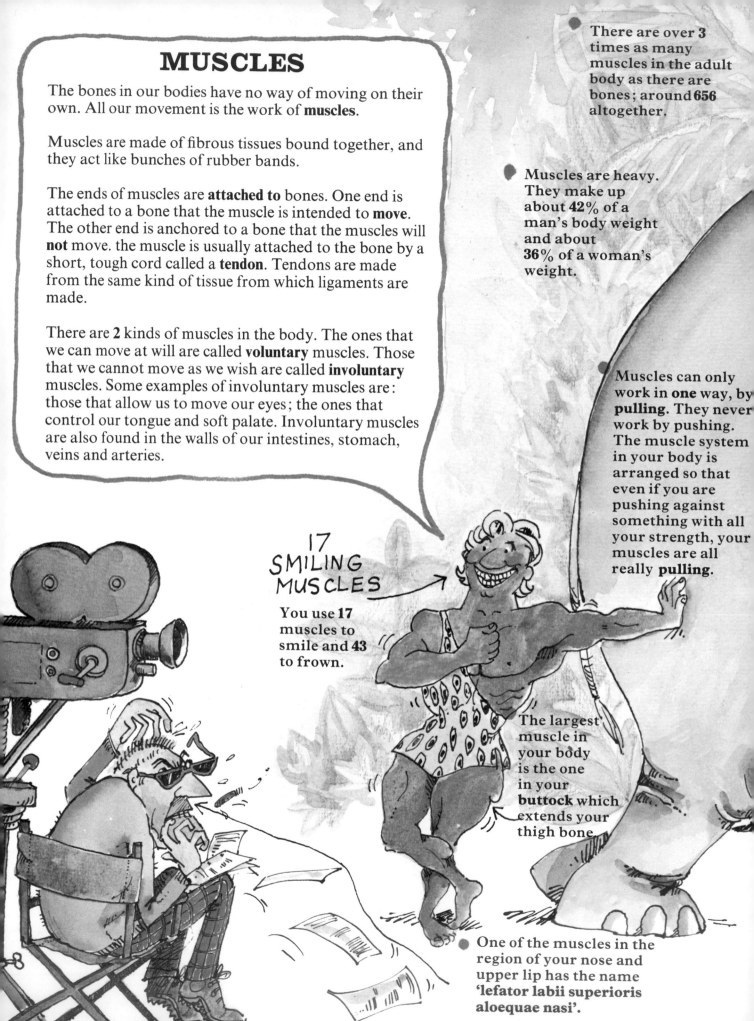

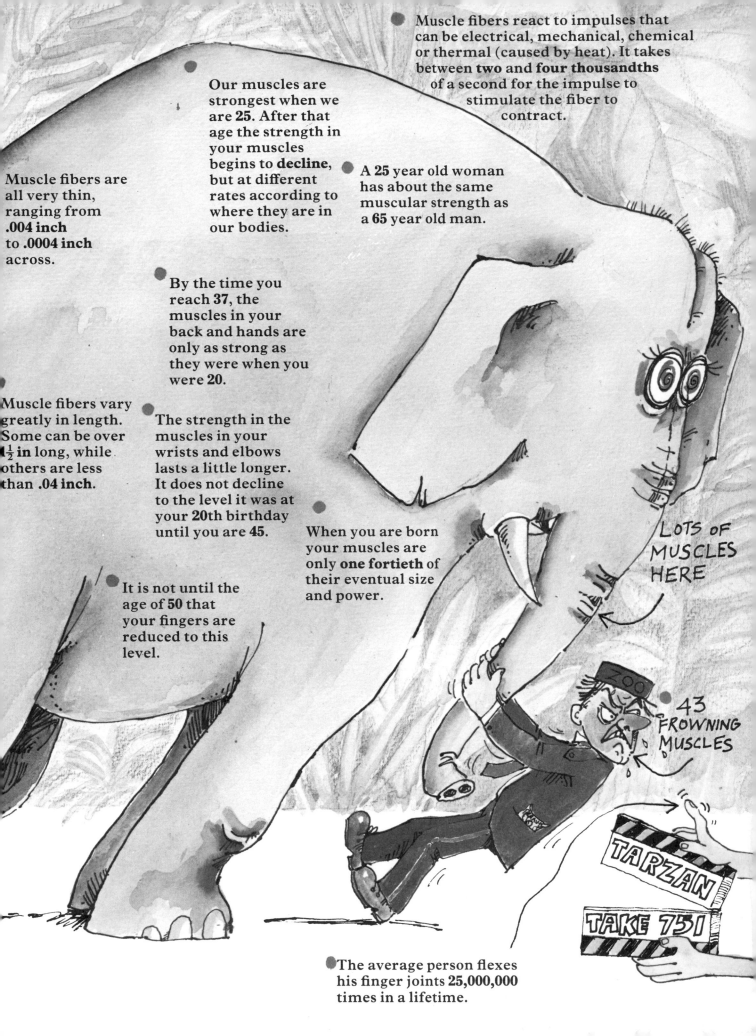

Muscle fibers react to impulses that can be electrical, mechanical, chemical or thermal (caused by heat). It takes between **two** and **four thousandths** of a second for the impulse to stimulate the fiber to contract.

Our muscles are strongest when we are **25**. After that age the strength in your muscles begins to **decline**, but at different rates according to where they are in our bodies.

A **25** year old woman has about the same muscular strength as a **65** year old man.

Muscle fibers are all very thin, ranging from **.004 inch** to **.0004 inch** across.

By the time you reach **37**, the muscles in your back and hands are only as strong as they were when you were **20**.

Muscle fibers vary greatly in length. Some can be over $1\frac{1}{2}$ **in** long, while others are less than **.04 inch**.

The strength in the muscles in your wrists and elbows lasts a little longer. It does not decline to the level it was at your **20th** birthday until you are **45**.

When you are born your muscles are only **one fortieth** of their eventual size and power.

It is not until the age of **50** that your fingers are reduced to this level.

LOTS OF MUSCLES HERE

43 FROWNING MUSCLES

ZOO

TARZAN

TAKE 751

The average person flexes his finger joints **25,000,000** times in a lifetime.

THE HEART

The heart is a **pump** that moves blood through the body. The blood is carried **away** from the heart in elastic tubes called **arteries** and it **returns** to the heart in elastic tubes called **veins**.

Together the heart, the blood, arteries and veins form what is known as the **circulatory system**.

Blood carries oxygen and other important materials to every part of the body through a mass of tiny arteries called **capillary arteries**. These capillary arteries are the finest tubes which connect arteries to veins. Through them the blood gives its nourishment to the body and also collects waste products like carbon dioxide, which it takes away.

The heart is, in fact, **2 pumps**. One pump receives blood **from the body** and sends it out to the lungs. The other pump receives blood **from the lungs** and sends it round the body.

The heart is divided into **4** chambers. The left and right side do **not** communicate. The upper chambers, known as **altria**, have quite thin walls and receive blood from the veins. The lower chambers are called **ventricles**. Blood carrying oxygen from the lungs enters the **left** atrium. Blood that has deposited its oxygen throughout the body enters the **right** atrium.

Both atria open into their corresponding ventricles through large **apertures** (openings). These apertures are guarded by **valves** that allow the blood to flow **one** way, but **not back up again**.

When we measure or feel our pulse, what we sense is not the actual arrival of blood at that pressure point, but a **ripple** over the surface of the arteries, which travels at about **23 feet per second**.

The blood in the arteries only travels at about **1.6 feet** per second.

The heart of a 47 year old man will have pumped a total **300,000 tons** of blood during his lifetime.

Strips of heart muscle will **continue to beat** even when they are isolated in a solution of warm saline (salt solution).

When you are **20** your heart will be pumping twice as much blood at one time as it will pump when you are **90** years old.

Every day the adult heart pumps blood through a total of about **155 miles** of blood vessels. That amount of pumping would be enough to fill a **4,630 gallon** tank.

The heart beat may rise to 100 or more beats a minute during exercise, so that the output of blood may be more than **21 quarts** a minute.

Vein

Right atrium

Right ventricle

LIVER

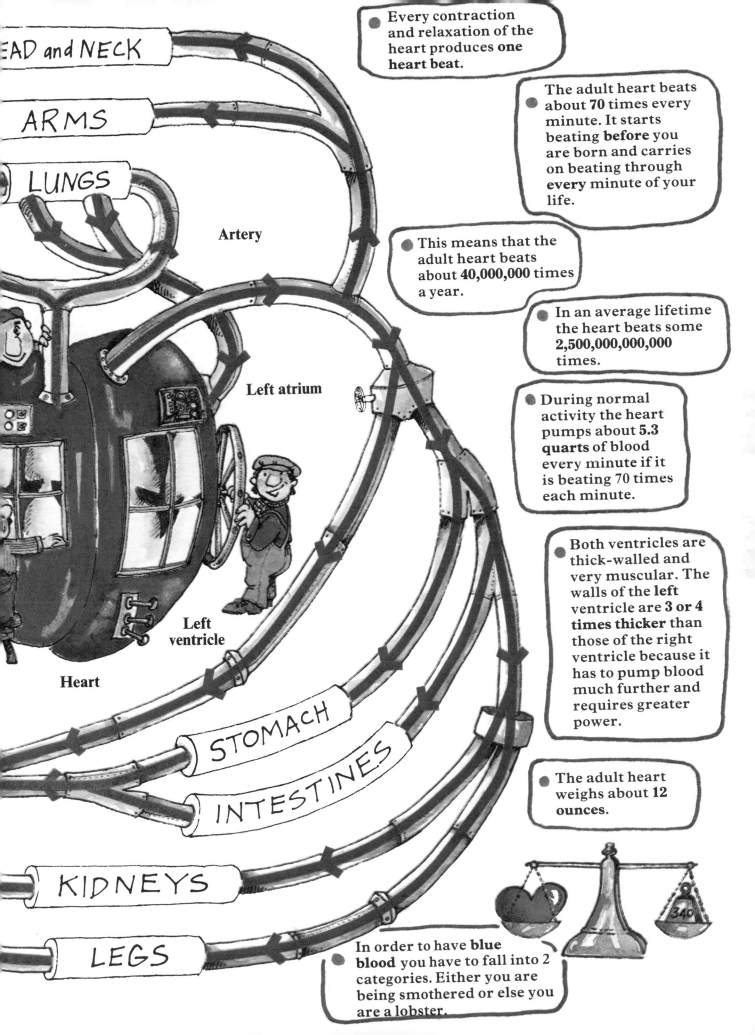

EAD and NECK

ARMS

LUNGS

Artery

Left atrium

Left ventricle

Heart

STOMACH

INTESTINES

KIDNEYS

LEGS

● Every contraction and relaxation of the heart produces **one heart beat.**

● The adult heart beats about **70** times every minute. It starts beating **before** you are born and carries on beating through **every** minute of your life.

● This means that the adult heart beats about **40,000,000** times a year.

● In an average lifetime the heart beats some **2,500,000,000,000** times.

● During normal activity the heart pumps about **5.3 quarts** of blood every minute if it is beating 70 times each minute.

● Both ventricles are thick-walled and very muscular. The walls of the **left ventricle** are **3 or 4 times thicker** than those of the right ventricle because it has to pump blood much further and requires greater power.

● The adult heart weighs about **12 ounces.**

● In order to have **blue blood** you have to fall into 2 categories. Either you are being smothered or else you are a lobster.

BLOOD

Blood is made up of a mixture of a liquid called **plasma** and **solids** called **red cells, white cells** and **platelets**.

Red cells are shaped like discs with a shallow depression on each side. They are very very small. The red cells are made in the red bone marrow of short bones like the breastbone, ribs and vertebrae. They take about **7 days** to form. Red cells are important because they contain a substance called **hemoglobin**. Hemoglobin **picks up oxygen** in the lungs and **carries it** to the tissues all over the body.

There are far fewer **white cells** but most of them are bigger than red cells. Their main job is to **combat harmful bacteria. Unlike red cells they have no** fixed shape, and they move about by changing shape.

The **platelets** are tiny oval structures (seen under a microscope). They are important in helping the blood to **clot**. If you cut yourself and there were no means by which your blood could clot, then all your blood would simply flow out. There are some people whose blood does not clot as quickly as most blood, and they have to be very careful not to injure themselves. The condition from which they suffer is known as **hemophilia**.

Plasma is **90%** water. The rest is made up of proteins and salts as well as waste products that are being carried round the circulatory system

Red Blood Cells

- Plasma is the color of straw and represents about **55%** of the total volume of our blood.

- The other **45%** is made up of: 25,000,000,000,000 red cells; up to 20,000,000,000 white cells; and 1,250,000,000,000 platelets.

- In terms of chemical composition the substance that most resembles human blood is **sea water**.

- When you are at rest, it takes about **6 seconds** for blood to be pumped from the heart to the lungs and back again.

- The journey to the brain and back again takes **8 seconds**. Pumping blood down to your toes and back to the heart again, takes **16 seconds**.

- The average man has **5-7 quarts** of blood in his body. The average woman has about **one quart less.**

- There are **valves** in our veins which stop all our blood rushing down to our legs when we stand up.

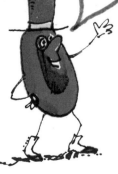

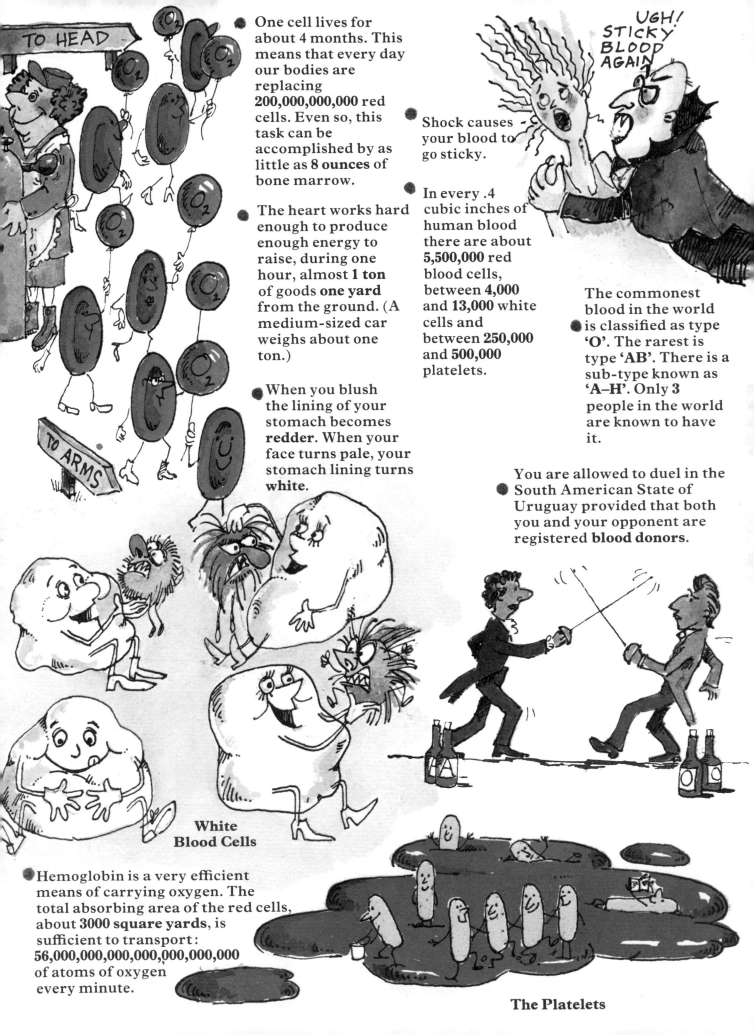

TO HEAD

One cell lives for about 4 months. This means that every day our bodies are replacing 200,000,000,000 red cells. Even so, this task can be accomplished by as little as **8 ounces** of bone marrow.

The heart works hard enough to produce enough energy to raise, during one hour, almost **1 ton** of goods **one yard** from the ground. (A medium-sized car weighs about one ton.)

When you blush the lining of your stomach becomes **redder**. When your face turns pale, your stomach lining turns **white**.

TO ARMS

Shock causes your blood to go sticky.

In every .4 cubic inches of human blood there are about **5,500,000** red blood cells, between **4,000** and **13,000** white cells and between **250,000** and **500,000** platelets.

UGH! STICKY BLOOD AGAIN

The commonest blood in the world is classified as type 'O'. The rarest is type 'AB'. There is a sub-type known as 'A–H'. Only **3** people in the world are known to have it.

You are allowed to duel in the South American State of Uruguay provided that both you and your opponent are registered **blood donors**.

White Blood Cells

Hemoglobin is a very efficient means of carrying oxygen. The total absorbing area of the red cells, about **3000 square yards**, is sufficient to transport: 56,000,000,000,000,000,000,000,000 of atoms of oxygen every minute.

The Platelets

THE BREATHING SYSTEM

Oxygen is distributed round the body by the blood which is pumped through the circulatory system by the heart. However the oxygen is absorbed into the bloodstream in the **lungs** and it enters the lungs as a result of a process we call **breathing**.

Air is constantly **drawn into** and **expelled from** the lungs by successive **changes in pressure** in the chest. These changes in pressure are brought about by a powerful, flat muscle called the **diaphragm, which lies across the body cavity.**

When the muscle moves **down** it causes the ribs to move **up** and **out**. This produces a **vacuum** in the lungs, which causes the outside pressure to force air **into the lungs** through the nose, throat and finally a tube called the **trachea**.

In the lungs an **exchange of gases** takes place. Some of the waste carbon-dioxide, brought from the body tissues by the blood, is released, and the blood absorbs some of the oxygen which has been brought in with the air.

This exchange of gas takes place in what are called **alveoli**. These are grape-like bunches of tiny **air-sacks**, each of which is covered in a cob-web of very fine capillaries. The red blood cells pass along these capillaries in **single file** and as they do, they **deposit** the carbon-dioxide they are carrying and **pick up** a supply of oxygen through the thin capillary wall.

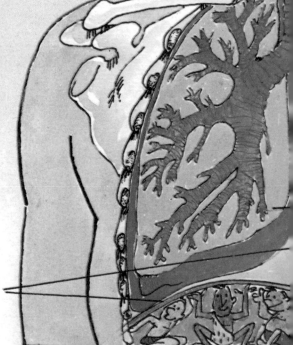

When you breathe gently through your nose, the **wind speed is 6.6 feet per second,** the same as a gentle breeze.

Your nose cleans, humidifies and **warms over 18.5 cubic yards** of air a day.

Diaphragm

A sneeze can travel fast as **100 miles per hour,** the speed of a hurricane.

ACH CHOOOO

100 M.P.H.

Laughing and **crying** are caused by very similar actions; a deep breathing in, followed by a series of short, sudden breathings out.

The **brain** requires **25%** of all the oxygen used by the body. The **kidneys** use **12%** and the **heart 7%**.

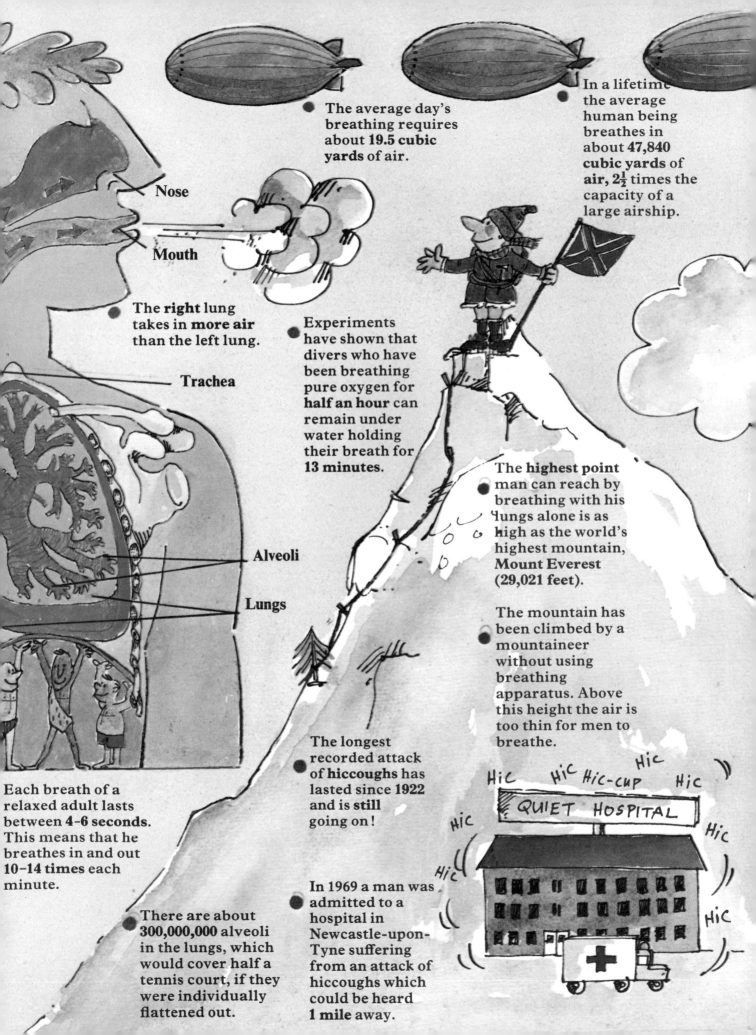

The average day's breathing requires about **19.5 cubic yards** of air.

In a lifetime the average human being breathes in about **47,840 cubic yards** of **air**, $2\frac{1}{2}$ times the capacity of a large airship.

Nose

Mouth

The **right** lung takes in **more air** than the left lung.

Trachea

Experiments have shown that divers who have been breathing pure oxygen for **half an hour** can remain under water holding their breath for **13 minutes.**

The **highest point** man can reach by breathing with his lungs alone is as high as the world's highest mountain, **Mount Everest (29,021 feet).**

Alveoli

Lungs

The mountain has been climbed by a mountaineer without using breathing apparatus. Above this height the air is too thin for men to breathe.

Each breath of a relaxed adult lasts between **4–6 seconds.** This means that he breathes in and out **10–14 times** each minute.

The longest recorded attack of **hiccoughs** has lasted since **1922** and is **still** going on!

Hic Hic Hic-cup Hic Hic
Hic

QUIET HOSPITAL

Hic
Hic
Hic

There are about **300,000,000** alveoli in the lungs, which would cover half a tennis court, if they were individually flattened out.

In 1969 a man was admitted to a hospital in Newcastle-upon-Tyne suffering from an attack of hiccoughs which could be heard **1 mile** away.

EATING

In order to be of any value to the body, the **food** which we eat must **enter** the **bloodstream** and be **distributed** to the tissues **throughout the body**.

Large pieces of insoluble food are **broken down** into smaller compounds. These smaller, soluble compounds pass through the walls of a length of tube called the **intestine**, to eventually enter the bloodstream. The process of breaking down insoluble food is called **digestion**.

Both digestion and absorption of food take place in a **muscular tube** which runs from the mouth to the anus. This tube is called the **alimentary canal**. The process of digesting the food is brought about by chemical compounds called **enzymes**.

As the food passes along the alimentary canal, it is **broken down in stages** by the **digestive juices**, which are introduced at different sections. The food which cannot be digested is **expelled**, with other waste products, through the **anus**.

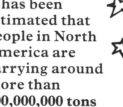

1. **Teeth**—cut and grind the food into small pieces.

2. **Cut Up Food**—is mixed with flui called saliva.

7. **Churned-up Food**—every 20 seconds waves pass through the stomach churning up the food and gastric juice into creamy fluid called **chyme**.

- Our food consists of elements called proteins, fats, carbohydrates, salts, vitamins and water. We need some of **all of these** to live.

- A man is claimed to have survived for **360 days** on a diet of **tap water**.

- While we are sleeping at night, we lose an average of **11 ounces** of weight.

- The desire to doze after a meal is caused by **chemicals** in the food itself.

- Food is measured according to the amount of **energy** it produces. The unit used to measure this energy is the **Calorie**.

- You need about **1 Calorie** of energy to read **650 words**. You need to eat a tomato or drink a cup of black coffee to get this energy.

- Roller skating uses from **200–500** Calories per hour.

- During our lifetime we eat about **60,000 pounds** of food, about the combined weight of **6** elephants.

- It has been estimated that people in North America are carrying around more than **200,000,000 tons** of excess fat.

- The **liver** is the **largest** gland in the body.

- Scientists have counted **500** functions of the liver. It is often called the body's chemical factory.

- If all the tiny tubes in the liver were laid end to end, they would stretch over **60 miles**.

9. **Semi-digested Food**—moves alon about **.8 inches** a second. It is churned up as it moves.

10. **Small Intestine: Ileum**—about **10** feet long. Most of t digestible food nov **soluble** compound which pass through the lining of the intestine into the bloodstream.

11. **Large Intestine: Colon**—here much of the water is extracted from the undigested matter and passed back into the bloodstream. This stops us becoming **dehydrated** (dried out).

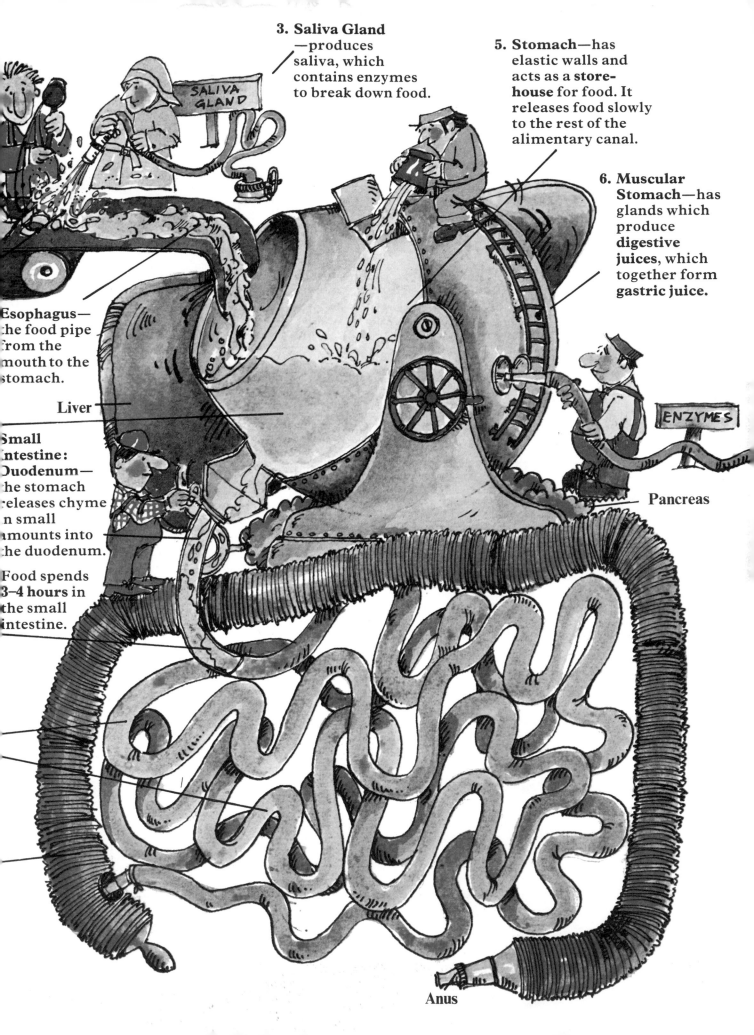

3. Saliva Gland
—produces saliva, which contains enzymes to break down food.

5. Stomach—has elastic walls and acts as a **storehouse** for food. It releases food slowly to the rest of the alimentary canal.

6. Muscular Stomach—has glands which produce **digestive juices**, which together form **gastric juice.**

SALIVA GLAND

Esophagus— the food pipe from the mouth to the stomach.

Liver

Small Intestine: Duodenum— the stomach releases chyme in small amounts into the duodenum.

Food spends **3–4 hours** in the small intestine.

ENZYMES

Pancreas

Anus

THE BRAIN AND THE NERVOUS SYSTEM

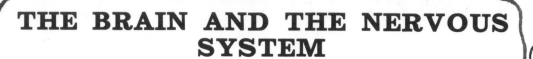

Eating our food involves a series of operations that are related to each other in time and space. Our eyes register that there is food on the plate. Our hands move to the right positions to pick it up. We raise the food to our mouths which open at just the right time to allow us to put the food inside and start chewing it. At the same time our mouths start to secrete saliva, beginning the digestive process. At the moment of swallowing the food, the other processes are brought into operation, and the food passes through the alimentary canal as a result of a series of controlled movements.

All these bodily functions are brought into operation at the right time as a result of **co-ordination**. Without co-ordination, eating would be **chaotic**. Eating is only one of the vast range of activities undertaken by our bodies. They **seem** automatic, but they are brought about by co-ordination, which is controlled by the **brain and the nervous system**.

The **brain**, is not part of a person, it is the person, his personality, his reactions, his mental capacity. The brain is the body's computer, constantly **receiving information** from inside and outside the body, constantly processing that information, acting as a result of it, and recording it for future reference. The brain is the **communications center** of a huge, intricate communications network which extends throughout the body along our nerves.

Only **one** person in every million has an IQ over 180.

Scientists have estimated that the speed of thought is only about **150 miles per hour**.

Impulses travel along our nerves about **20 miles per hour** faster than the world helicopter speed record.

The human brain does **not** feel pain. Headaches originat from the muscles a nerves surrounding the brain.

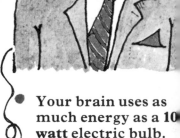

Your brain uses as much energy as a 10 **watt** electric bulb.

The brain requires constant supplies of oxygen, blood and glucose. **20%** of the oxygen we breathe in and **15%** of our blood goes to the brain.

The human brain is a **4.8 ounce** mushroom of grey and white tissue wit the consistency of je

The nerve network in your brain contains more possib connections than there would be in a universal telephone exchange, which supplied a telephone to every person on Earth.

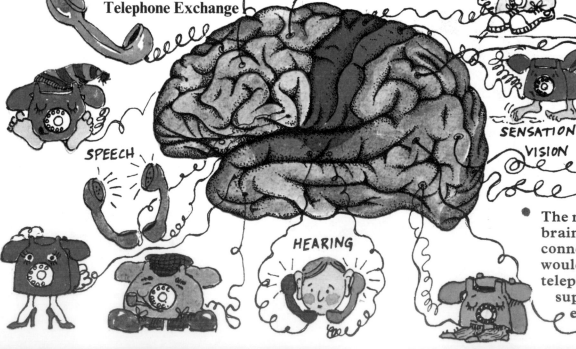

The Brain as a Telephone Exchange

SPEECH

HEARING

SENSATION

VISION

There are nearly **45 miles** of nerves running through our bodies.

The basic units of the nervous system are nerve cells called **neurons**.

A Motor Nerve

The **central nervous system** is connected to **every** part of the body by **43 pairs** of nerves. **12 pairs** go to and from the brain, and **31** go from the spinal cord.

The nerves form an **intricate network** that extends from your toenails to the roots of the hair on your head.

● There are up to **1,300** nerve endings in every **square inch** of our hands.

Messages travel along the nerves as **electrical impulses**. The fastest they travel is about **248 miles per hour**. In the smaller nerves the speed is slower.

● The millions of nerve cells are **grouped** mainly into the **central nervous system**, the **brain** and the **spinal cord**.

● There are about **14,000,000,000** cells in the human brain.

The human brain is about **80% water**.

● The **right** side of the brain receives messages and controls the **left** side of the body.

Cross-section of the Brain

The brain has **3 sections**. The **2 hemispheres** form the **cerebrum** which controls learning, thinking and the memory.

At the back of the skull is the **cerebellum** which controls the muscles.

The **spinal cord** leaves the brain below the medulla and goes **4/5ths** of the way down the back. It is only $\frac{1}{2}$ **inch** wide, and weighs about **1 ounce**.

THUMP THUMP

The medulla controls the **automatic** bodily functions, like the action of the heart and the operation of the respiratory system. It is also the **main** sense center for senses like taste, balance, hearing and posture.

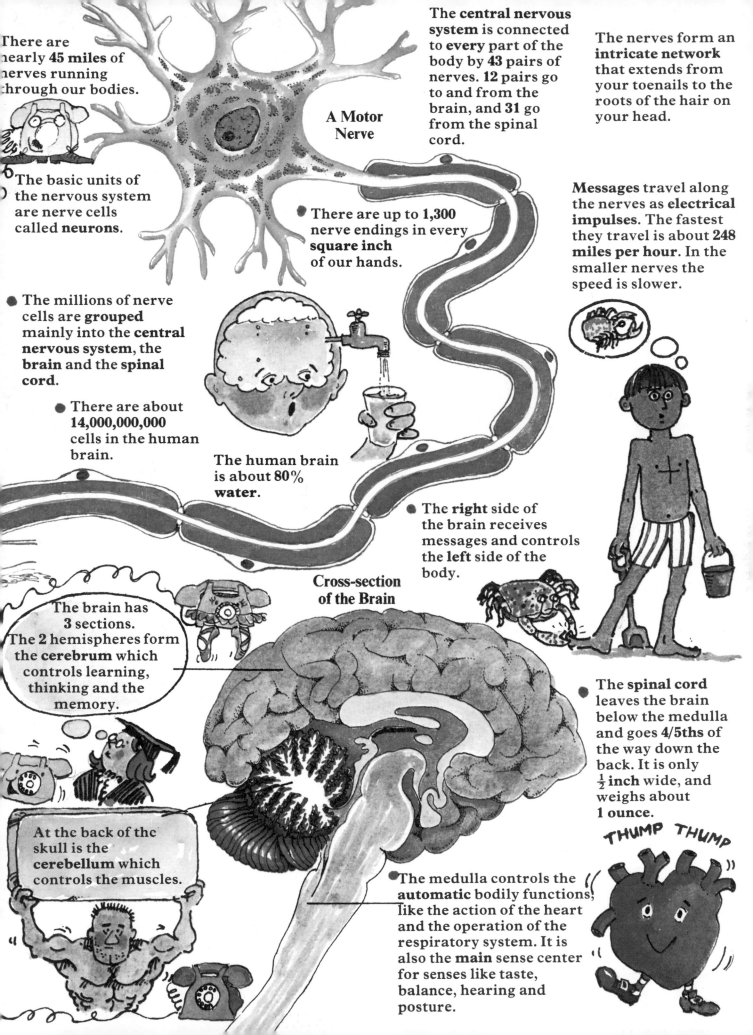

EYESIGHT

We all know that our eyes enable us to **see**, but how many of us realize how **complicated** this process is? The human eye is no larger than a **ping-pong ball**, yet it contains **tens of millions** of electrical connections, is able to handle **1,500,000** messages at the same time and gathers about **80%** of the knowledge we absorb.

The cells in the retina are so **sensitive** they can register light as dim as **1/100,000,000,000,000** of a watt. They are so sensitive that a person sitting on top of a mountain, on a clear night, with no moon, can see a match struck **50 miles** away.

Blue eyes are the **most** sensitive to light.

Brown eyes have **more pigment** (coloring matter) than blue eyes.

Retina—layer of cells which **respond to** light. There are 2 types of cells—**rods** and **cones**—depending on their shape. There are about **7,000,000** cones and **12,000,000** rods. Only cones see **color.**

Optic Nerve—made up of **800,000** nerve fibers. It **connects** the rods and cones in the retina to the brain.

When light passes through the lens it is turned **upside down** and **reversed** from left to right. The image is passed down the optic nerve like this until it reaches the brain, where it is **returned** to its real appearance.

Retina

Vitreous Humour— a clear jelly filling this large space.

Cross-section of the Eye

Cornea—the 'see-through' section.

Optic Nerve

Pupil—when **bright** light reaches the iris, the muscles contract and close up, and the pupil becomes **narrower**. When the light is **dim**, the muscles relax, and the pupil **expands** to let more light in.

Pupil

Each of your eyes sees a **different** picture, so your brain puts the **2** pictures together to get a **complete** image of what you are looking at.

Iris–colored part of the eye. Round its inner edge is a ring of tiny muscles sensitive to light.

Lens—made of strong **see-through** tissue. The shape can be **altered** by muscles attached to its rim so the lens can focus on things near or far from the eye.

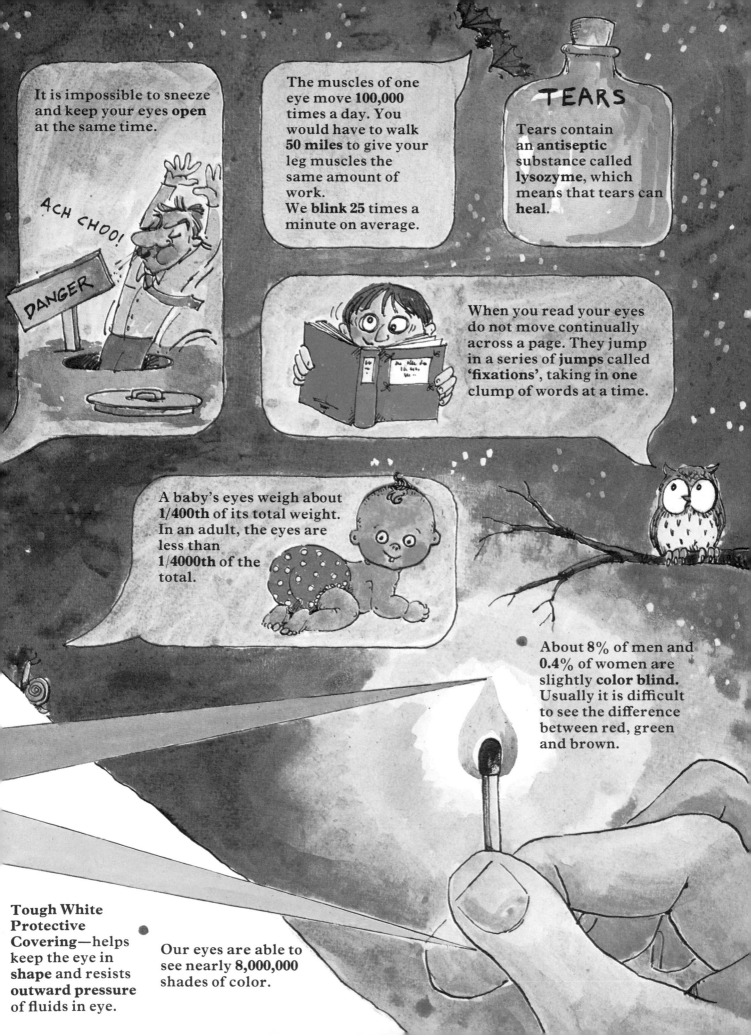

It is impossible to sneeze and keep your eyes **open** at the same time.

ACH CHOO!

DANGER

The muscles of one eye move **100,000** times a day. You would have to walk **50 miles** to give your leg muscles the same amount of work.
We **blink 25** times a minute on average.

TEARS

Tears contain an **antiseptic** substance called **lysozyme**, which means that tears can **heal**.

When you read your eyes do not move continually across a page. They jump in a series of **jumps** called **'fixations'**, taking in **one** clump of words at a time.

A baby's eyes weigh about **1/400th** of its total weight. In an adult, the eyes are less than **1/4000th** of the total.

About **8%** of men and **0.4%** of women are slightly **color blind**. Usually it is difficult to see the difference between red, green and brown.

Tough White Protective Covering—helps keep the eye in **shape** and resists **outward pressure** of fluids in eye.

Our eyes are able to see nearly **8,000,000** shades of color.

Outer-Ear— sound passes from here down the passage lined with **thousands** of **hairs** and **4,000 wax glands.**

Hair and Wax Gland—**clean** the air of dust and other particles. They clean dirty water when we put our heads under water.

Ear-drum—closes the end of the passage. It is tightly-stretched membrane, about **one half inch** across.

Outer E

The sound-bearing airwaves strike the membrane, like a drum, and it **vibrates.**

Passage

HEARING AND EARS

Our **ears** are not simply pieces of skin sticking out of the sides of our heads. Each one is filled with **vital miniaturized sensory equipment**, packed into a space not much bigger than a **hazelnut**.

The flap of skin and tissue on the outside is really a **trumpet** which gathers the sound into the ear and enables it to be channeled down a passage about **1 inch** long **into our heads**. At the end of the passage is the **inner ear**, where all the important work of the ear is performed. Inside this small space there are enough electrical circuits to provide a telephone service for a good-sized city.

Although we think that the main function of our ears is to allow us to hear, this is only **part** of the ears' function.

The inner ear is filled with **3** distinct sensory systems of which hearing is only one. The other **2** are organs of **balance** that allow us to stay **upright** and **warn our brains** when we are about to fall over. These organs of balance also enable us to judge the **movements** of **turning our heads** so that we maintain our balance when we move our heads about.

Sound intensity is measured in **decibels**. A normal conversation = **about 60**; a loud shout = **about 90**; a pop group's sound = **about 120**; a gunshot = **about 140.**

A dog can distinguish sounds **11°** apart. Humans can only hear sounds **45°** apart.

The sounds which carry **best** and are **easiest** for the human ear to hear are, "ah", "aw", "eh", "ee" and "oo".

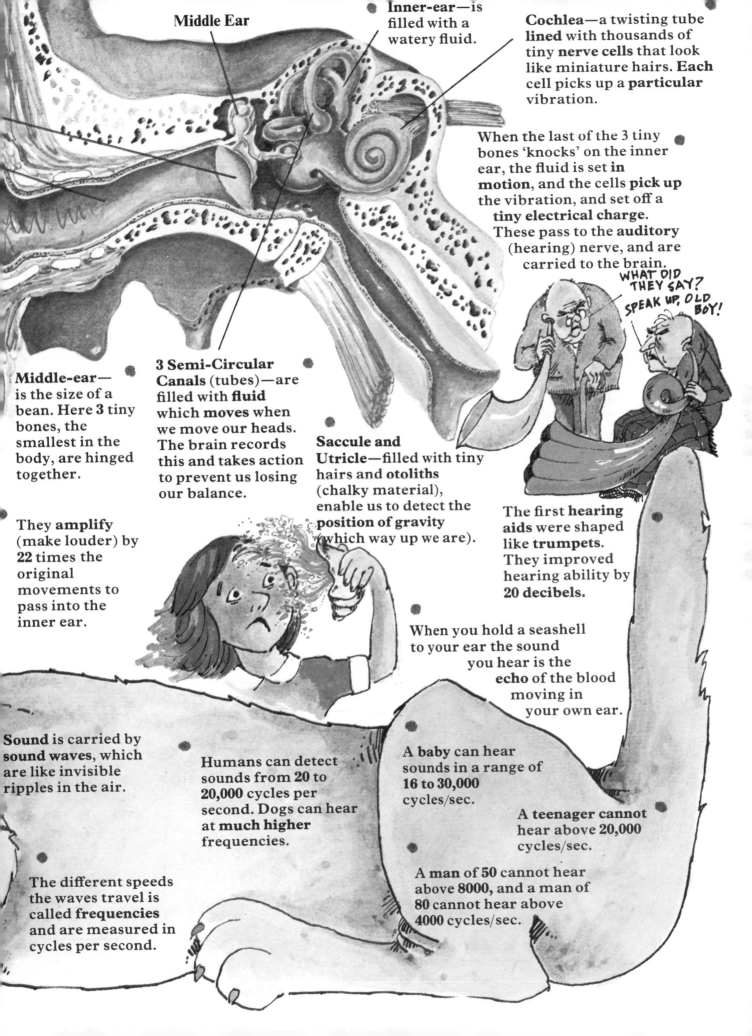

Middle Ear

Inner-ear—is filled with a watery fluid.

Cochlea—a twisting tube **lined** with thousands of tiny **nerve cells** that look like miniature hairs. **Each** cell picks up a **particular** vibration.

When the last of the 3 tiny bones 'knocks' on the inner ear, the fluid is set **in motion**, and the cells **pick up** the vibration, and set off a **tiny electrical charge**. These pass to the **auditory** (hearing) nerve, and are carried to the brain.

WHAT DID THEY SAY? SPEAK UP, OLD BOY!

Middle-ear— is the size of a bean. Here **3** tiny bones, the smallest in the body, are hinged together.

3 Semi-Circular Canals (tubes)—are filled with **fluid** which **moves** when we move our heads. The brain records this and takes action to prevent us losing our balance.

Saccule and Utricle—filled with tiny hairs and **otoliths** (chalky material), enable us to detect the **position of gravity** (which way up we are).

The first **hearing aids** were shaped like **trumpets**. They improved hearing ability by **20 decibels.**

They **amplify** (make louder) by **22** times the original movements to pass into the inner ear.

When you hold a seashell to your ear the sound you hear is the **echo** of the blood moving in your own ear.

Sound is carried by **sound waves**, which are like invisible ripples in the air.

Humans can detect sounds from 20 to 20,000 cycles per second. Dogs can hear at **much higher** frequencies.

A baby can hear sounds in a range of **16** to **30,000** cycles/sec.

A teenager cannot hear above 20,000 cycles/sec.

A man of 50 cannot hear above **8000**, and a man of **80** cannot hear above **4000** cycles/sec.

The different speeds the waves travel is called **frequencies** and are measured in cycles per second.

TASTE AND . . .

There are **4** primary sensations of taste—swee[t] bitter, sour and salt. These are identified by **taste receptors** in the **taste buds** on the **upper** surface of the tongue. Not all taste buds are o[n] the tongue though. There are some on the **palate** and some at the **top** of the **throat** on the **pharynx** and **tonsils**.

TOO SALTY   TOO SWEET

MMMMM

SLURP

YUM YUM!

YUM YUM!

Your tongue **print** is as **unique** as your finger print.

The ability to taste sweet things **decreases** as we get older.
You lose your sense of smell **sooner** than any of the other 4 senses.

Nothing solid can be tasted unless part of it can be **dissolved** in saliva on the tongue.

A man's tongue weighs about **2 ounces** and is about **4 inch** long.

New-born babies have taste buds **all over** the insides of their mouths. By the time they are adults only the ones in their tongues and throats are left.

BITTER

SALT

SOUR

SWEET

Different tastes are detected by **different** taste buds, which are on **different parts** of the tongue.
The taste buds at the **tip** detect sweetness; the ones at the **side**, sourness; the ones near the **base**, bitterness; ones at the **side** and at the **tip**, saltiness.

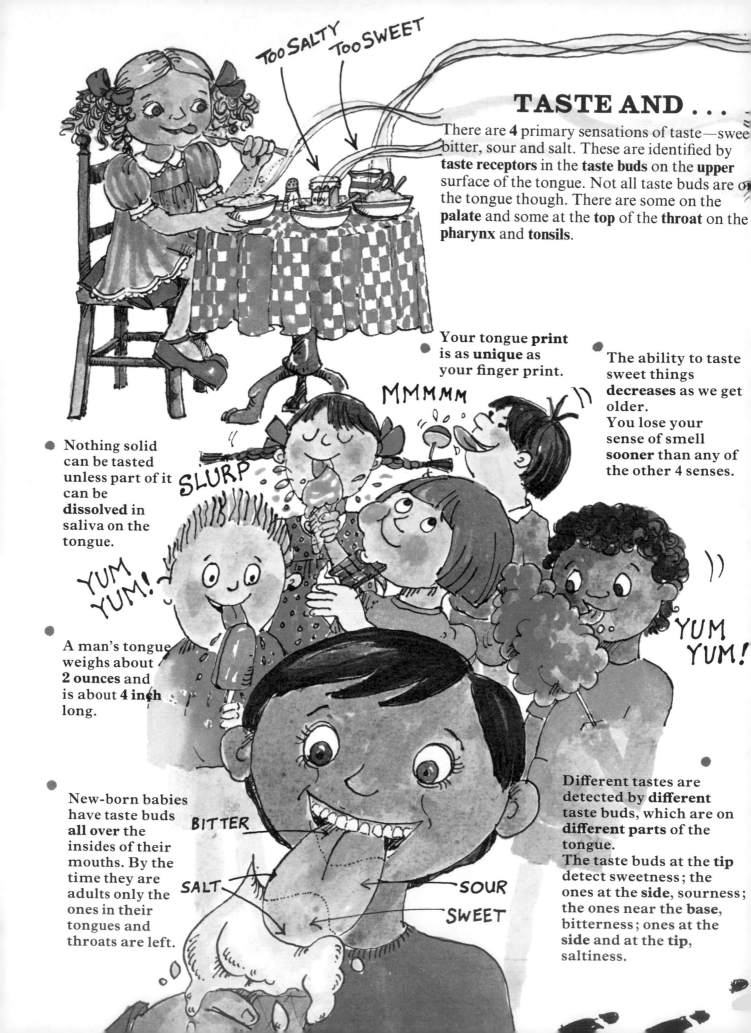

SMELL

Unlike the receptors that sense taste, which are grouped into about **9000** taste buds, the several million receptors that detect smell are distributed fairly **evenly** over the roof of each of the **nasal cavities** (in the nose). From **each** of these cells **6–8** tiny sensory hairs project. **Each** of the receptory cells is **connected with the brain**, about **1 inch** away. **Signals** pass from the cells to the brain which converts them into the sense we call **odors** and **smells**.

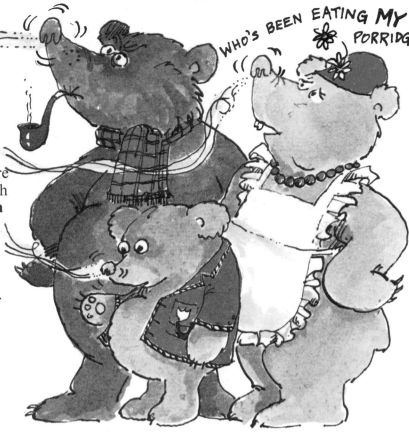

WHO'S BEEN EATING MY PORRIDGE?

A NOSE FOR A ROSE

All odors have to be dissolved in **mucus** in the **olfactory** (smelling) organs before they can be detected by the sensory cells in the nasal cavities.

It used to be believed that the mucus which flows down your nose when you have a cold, was fluid flowing **out of your brain**.

Most people are able to distinguish **4000** different smells. Really sensitive noses can distinguish about **10,000**.

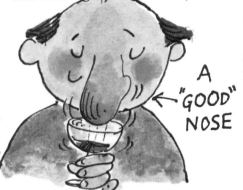

A "GOOD" NOSE

When dogs follow a man's trail they follow the scent he leaves in each of his **footprints**.

A dog can detect **one millionth** of that amount, and so can follow **old** scents.

Scientists have estimated that about **250,000,000,000** molecules of the smelly substance in sweat is deposited in each footprint.

Even a **man** can follow a fresh human trail, if it has been left on a firm floor, and if he is prepared to go down on all fours and sniff.

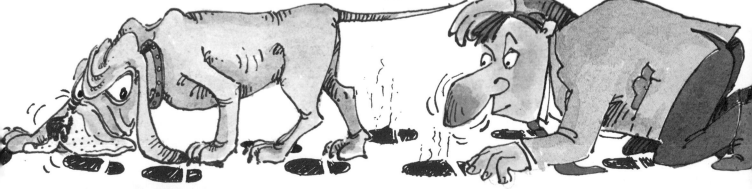

TEETH

Most human babies are born with no visible teeth. The **first** teeth normally appear between the ages of **5½ to 10 months** and **continue** to appear until the child is **27** months old. It then has a **full set** of **20 deciduous** or **milk teeth**. These milk teeth are **replaced** as the child gets older with **32 permanent** teeth that are designed to last the rest of the child's life.

There were **10 badly decayed teeth found in the skull of Zimbabwe Man**. Zimbabwe Man was one of the **earliest** men to live on Earth.

A total of 4 tons of decayed teeth are pulled from the mouths of children in England and Wales every year.

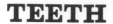

INCISORS

CANINES

MOLARS

Most of a tooth is made up of **2** substances.
1—enamel, the 'skin' of the tooth, is the **hardest tissue** in the human body. It is **96%** mineral.
2—dentine—is the **inner** part of the tooth, similar to bone, but harder.

A complete set of adult teeth consists of: **8 incisors**, cutting teeth; **20 molars** that grind the food cut by the incisors; **4 canines** which help to cut up the food.

Although it is possible to **transplant** teeth, they tend to **fall** out after a few years.

Brushing with **salt** cleans teeth as effectively as brushing with toothpaste.

British children from **5–17** have about $9\frac{1}{2}$ **million** fillings in their teeth each year. $1\frac{1}{2}$ **million** teeth are removed.

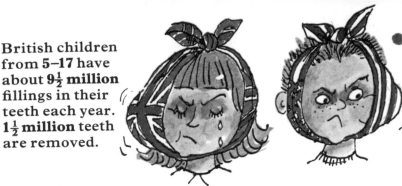

Official figures in the U.S.A. show that **97%** of American children suffer from some form of tooth decay.

Many people wear false teeth which contain a minute amount of **radioactive uranium** to stimulate fluorescence. It prevents the false teeth looking **dull green** in artificial light.

Fudge and **plain chocolate** are the foods **most** likely to give you tooth decay.

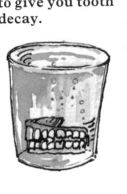

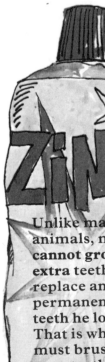

Doughnuts are among the **least** harmful of the sweet foods.

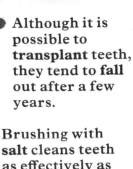

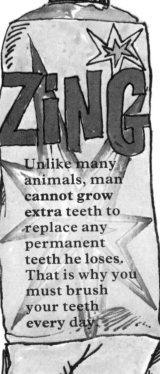

ZiNG

Unlike many animals, man **cannot grow extra** teeth to replace any permanent teeth he loses. That is why you must brush your teeth every day.

HAIR AND NAILS

Hairs are some of the **fastest** growing tissues in the human body, which is surprising because hairs are **dead.** It is the root of the hair which is living and this pushes up the hair cells through the skin. The name of the hair root is the **follicle.**

The hair in a man's beard is about as **tough** as **copper wire** of the same thickness.

Every year a man produces about **5.6 inches** of beard and the hairs on his scalp grow about **5 inches** in the same time. It would take about **6** years to grow hair long enough to sit on.

Human hair and nails do **not** continue to grow after death. They are the **last** part of the body to disintegrate.

It is possible to **transplant** fingernails.

If you are left-handed the nails on your **left** hand will grow **faster** than those on your right hand and vice versa.

Fingernails grow at a rate of **0.02 inch** per week.

The nail on your **middle** finger grows **faster** than all the other nails.

OH RAPUNZEL, RAPUNZEL, LET DOWN YOUR HAIR

Hair follicles work day and night for at least **3** years before they shut down for 3 or 4 months for a **rest.**

During this rest the old hair **falls out**, but once the follicle starts up again, the hair grows once more.

The **curliness** of a hair is determined by the shape of its **cross-section.** **Straight** hair has a circular cross-section; **wavy** hair, elliptical; **curly** hair has kidney-shaped cross-section.

On average we **lose** between **30** and **60** individual hairs every day.

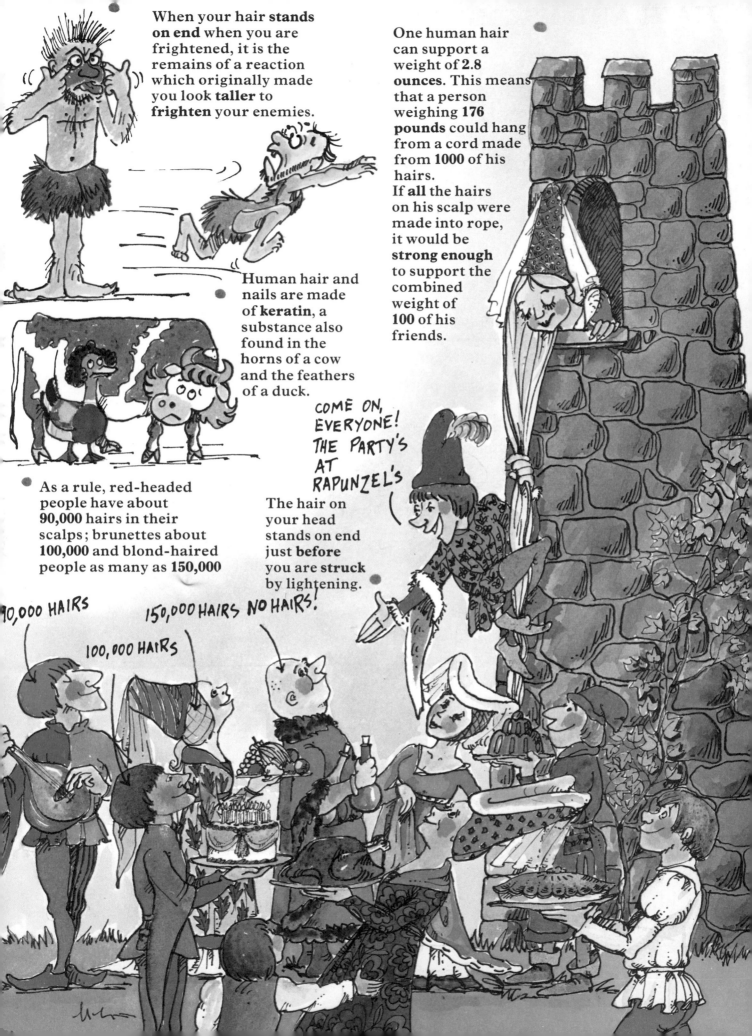

When your hair **stands on end** when you are frightened, it is the remains of a reaction which originally made you look **taller** to **frighten** your enemies.

Human hair and nails are made of **keratin**, a substance also found in the horns of a cow and the feathers of a duck.

One human hair can support a weight of **2.8 ounces**. This means that a person weighing **176 pounds** could hang from a cord made from **1000** of his hairs.
If **all** the hairs on his scalp were made into rope, it would be **strong enough** to support the combined weight of **100** of his friends.

As a rule, red-headed people have about **90,000** hairs in their scalps; brunettes about **100,000** and blond-haired people as many as **150,000**

COME ON, EVERYONE! THE PARTY'S AT RAPUNZEL'S

The hair on your head stands on end just **before** you are **struck** by lightening.

90,000 HAIRS

100,000 HAIRS

150,000 HAIRS NO HAIRS!

SKIN

The **skin** provides far **more** functions than simply to provide a convenient **wrapper** for all the ingredients that make up the human body. The skin **manufactures** important **chemicals** like **Vitamin D**. It **keeps in** the body fluids without which we would quickly die and it **keeps out** excess water when we go swimming or sit in the bath for a long time. It is vital in **cooling** the body and in **conserving** its heat. It **forms** our shape. The complex nervous system **detects** pain, touch, heat and cold and instantly passes these findings on to the brain.

- The average adult has some **2,000,000** sweat glands in the **9.6 sq yd.** of skin covering his body.

- Each sweat gland is a tightly coiled **tube** buried deep inside the dermis, connected to the surface by a tube about **0.2 inch** long.

- There is a total length of about **5.9 miles** of these **ducts** (tubes) in the adult body.

WRONG SIZE SKIN!

- **One** wrinkle is produced by every **200,000** frowns.

- Every day **millions** of epidermal cells are **washed off** or **rubbed off** by the clothes we wear. This means we actually get a **new outer skin every 27** days.

The Chinese were using **fingerprints** as a means of legal identification in **AD 700**.

- There are **more** sweat glands in the **palms** of our hands and the **soles** of our feet than in any other part of our bodies.

- You can only receive a skin graft from another part of your **own** body or from the body of your **identical** twin.

- The sense of **touch** is really **5** sensations – touch, pressure, pain, heat and cold. Often these senses have **combined** nerve endings. The nerve endings that detect pain are most numerous; then comes touch, then heat and cold.

- It is **easier** to pinpoint the area of pain or touch than the point of heat or cold.

- Although the skin is generally **0.04–0.08 inch** thick, it is as little as **0.02 inch** thick over the eyelids, and as much as **0.24 inch** thick on the palms and soles of our feet.

- There is **less** water in fat than in any other tissue in the human body, including bone.

Cross-section of the Skin

The skin consists of **2 principle layers**—the **dermis** and the **epidermis**.

Epidermis—the outer layer is formed from cells constantly being pushed up towards the surface by a steady **replacement** from beneath.

By the time it reaches the surface, the cell is **dead**. It forms part of the **protective** surface before it is flaked off and replaced by another dead cell.

Hair

Hair root

Sweat Gland

Dermis—contains blood capillaries, nerve endings, fat cells, sweat glands, roots of hairs, erector muscles for each hair (which cause goose-pimples) and other loose connective tissue.

Subcutaneous fat—a layer of fat which acts as a **food reserve**, and as an **insulating** layer reducing heat loss.

● On the average, under $\frac{1}{5}$ **square inch** of skin there are:— about **100** sweat glands; **hundreds** of nerve endings; **11 feet** of nerves; **3 feet** of blood vessels; **10** hair follicles and **15 sebaceous** glands (that produce the oil in our hair).

In the palms of our hands there may be as many as **2906 sweat glands** in **every square inch**.

● Apart from being the **largest** organ in the human body, the skin also accounts for about **16**% of the total body weight.

If you sit in water for a long time, the skin on the soles of your feet and on your palms, **wrinkle**. This happens because these areas **lack** the glands that secrete fatty, lubricating substance which prevents the skin from absorbing water.

The amount of **sweat** we produce relates to how **hot** our bodies become. The average human being, doing light work, in a temperate climate, may lose **3.01 quart** a day. A miner may lose **7.82 quart**, and a worker in a hot climate, like India, can lose up to **12.04 quart** a day.

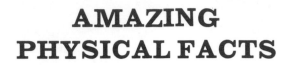

AMAZING PHYSICAL FACTS

The longest period in which a person has **yawned** continuously is **5 weeks**.

A Korean boy aged **4 years 8 months** appeared on Japanese television speaking **4** languages (Korean, English, German and Japanese), **composing poetry** and performing **integral calculus** (advanced mathematics).

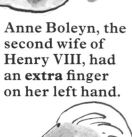

Anne Boleyn, the second wife of Henry VIII, had an **extra** finger on her left hand.

The average medieval man was only **5 feet 6 inches** tall and weighed **134 pounds**.

The Padaung people of Burma **extend** the length of their necks by fitting coils one above the other which stretches the neck and pushes the shoulders down over the years. The greatest recorded length is **15¾ inches**.

The first American President, George Washington, was one of the first men to wear **false teeth**. He had many sets, including one made from elm wood and another carved from hippopotamus ivory.

The BBC racing commentator, Raymond Glendenning, once spoke **176 words in 30 seconds** while he was giving a commentary on a greyhound race.

The **longest** finger nail officially measured was **24.9 inches** long.

An Italian dentist who **kept** all the teeth he extracted during his **36 years** in practice, had over **2,000,000** teeth.

Almost **half** the heat in your body is lost through the **top** of your head.

An Indian Brahmin has grown a moustache which has an extended span of **102 inches**.

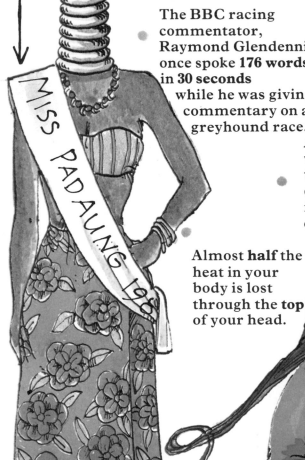

(15¾ inches)

MISS PADAUNG 19...

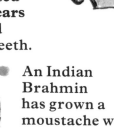

(102 inches)

ELM

The average life-span for cavemen was **18 years**. For ancient Romans the average was **22 years**. In 1850 the average in the civilized world was **37 years**. Today, in most industrialized nations, it has risen to over **70 years**.

The smallest waist measured in modern times is **13.0 inches**. In the 16th century, the French Queen, Catherine de Medici, decreed that women at the French court should have waists measuring **13.0 inches** as a matter of fashion.

The first Tzar of Russia, Peter The Great, decreed that there should be a **tax on beards** in his kingdom. Eventually he **banned** beards altogether.

(8 feet 11 inches)

Robert Wadlow, the **tallest** man ever measured, stood **8 ft 11 in** tall, had an arm span of **3.1 yds**, his feet were **18.8 inches** long and his hands were **12¾ inches** long.

When he was 21 he weighed **490 pounds**.

The Mbuti pygmies have an averge height of **4 feet 6 in** for men and **4 feet 4 in** for women.

The **longest** beard ever measured was grown by a Norwegian called Hans Langseth. At the time of his death his beard had grown to a length of **17.5 feet**.

(13 inches)

(4 foot 6 inches)

(12¾ inches)

(17½ feet)

(18½ inches)

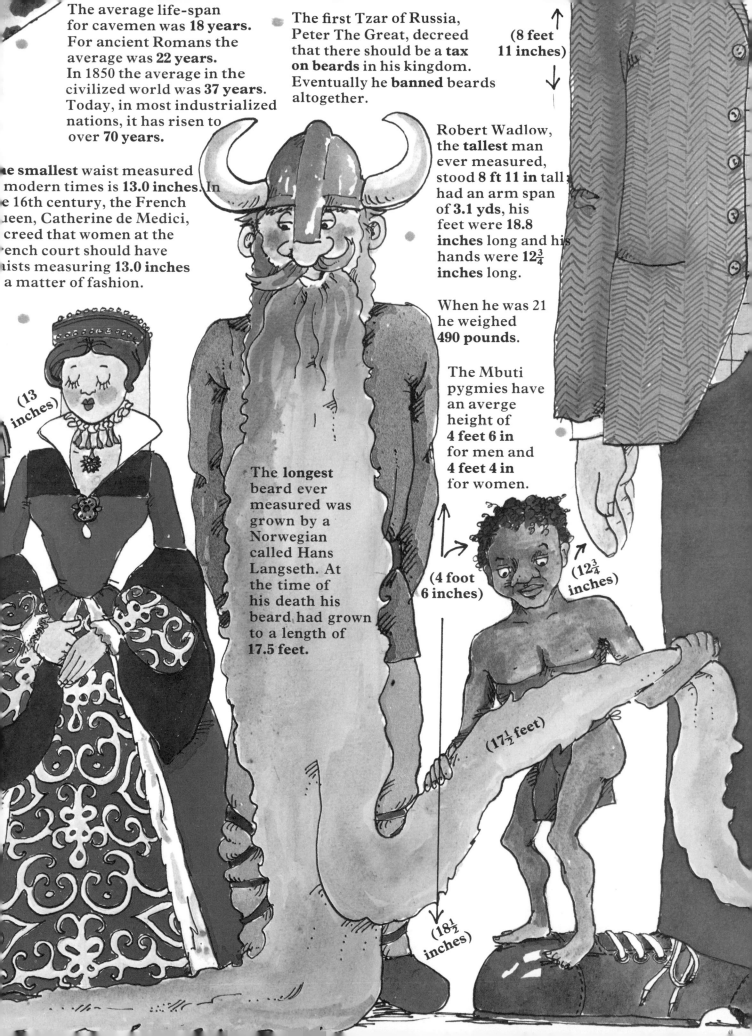

SUM TOTAL

An American scientist has calculated that it would **cost** about **$6,000,000** to manufacture the complicated proteins and enzymes in the human body. The estimated cost for producing human cells from these compounds is put at **$18,000,000,000** and the cost for actually assembling a human body from these cells was stated as being beyond **'human comprehension'**.

The average person weighing **150 pounds** contains about **143 pounds** of water, protein and stored fat. The rest of the weight is made up by acids, chemicals and minerals.

The average woman contains enough hydrogen to fill a balloon that would be able to lift her to the **top of Mt. Snowdon.**

There is enough iron in the body of a healthy adult to make **one nail 3 inches** long.

We each contain enough sulphur to **kill** all the fleas on a dog.

The lime in the human body would be enough to **white-wash** a small chicken-coop.

$\frac{2}{3}$ of the body's weight is **water**. If you drained all the water out of a man weighing **160 pounds** hi weight would be immediate **reduced to 66 pounds.**

A baby contains **more copper** in its liver and brain than an adult.

If all the phosphorous in the human body was used for making the heads of matches, there would be enough for **2,000** match-heads.

There is as much **carbon** in the human body as there is in the lead of **900 pencils.**

The **potassium** in the human body would be adequate to **explode** a toy **cannon.**

BACK

You could make **7 bars of soap** with the fat in the human body.

If all the bacteria living on our bodies could be collected, there would be enough to **fill a tea-cup**